How To Make A Baby
Proven Method That Shows Those Trying To Conceive How To Have A Baby Fast

Simone Novelette

All Rights Reserved. No part of this publication may be reproduced in any form or by any means, including scanning, photocopying, or otherwise without prior written permission of the copyright holder. Copyright © 2013

Table of Contents

1. Fertility Facts And The Effects Of Aging...4-9
2. The Ovulation and Menstrual Cycles...10-15
3. What To Avoid And What To Embrace When Trying To Conceive...16-22
4. Sexual Positions That Help You To Get Pregnant...23-25
5. Fertility Signs...26-29
6. The Natural Way To Find Out If You Ovulate...30-39
7. Find Out Exactly When You Ovulate...40-45
8. Selecting Your Baby's Gender...46-48
9. Am I Pregnant?...49-54
10. When Pregnancy Goes Wrong...55-60
11. Major Causes Of Female Infertility...61-73
12. Major Causes Of Male Infertility...74-79
13. Infertility Testing...80-83
14. Getting Help To Conceive...84-89

Chapter 1

Fertility Facts And The Effects Of Aging

There are several myths about fertility that continue to be thought of as the truth. Many people believe them and some of them actually do more harm than good to your dreams of conception, below the common myths are exposed so that you can begin to understand your body. Here are the facts:

1. Men have as much chance as women do of having fertility problems, in fact, 40% of the time, the male partner is the one whose fertility issues prevent a couple from conceiving.
2. All menstrual cycles are NOT 28 days long. Normal cycles may range from 24 to 36 days long.
3. All women do NOT ovulate on day 14 of their cycle. Women have been known to ovulate as early as Day 8 of their cycle.

4. A basal temperature rise does NOT mean you are at your fertile peak, in fact, it means the opposite. It indicates that you have ovulated and your egg is long gone.
5. Cervical fluid WILL give a firm indication of when you are nearing ovulation.
6. Women are not fertile all the time, it is men who are fertile all the time. A woman is only fertile on the day she ovulates and at least five days before ovulation. This is because sperm can survive for up to five days to implant the egg on the day of ovulation. Once ovulation is over, usually within 24hrs, a woman cannot get pregnant again that cycle.

Those are the facts, don't worry if at this point you don't understand clearly terms such as, cervical fluid and basal temperature, all of this will be explained later in the book. If you do understand what those terms mean then that is even better, but you will know more about them once you are finished with this book.

The Effects Of Aging On Female Fertility

There has always been much debate about the best age for a woman to have a baby. This depends on if you are looking at it from a financial point of view or a biological point of view. There is no doubt that the early twenties are the best time biologically for a woman to have a baby. However, these days women are busy going to college and getting an education. There are also many other personal reasons for delaying pregnancy, some women do not find a suitable partner until later in life. Whatever the reason for women getting pregnant later in life, it is becoming a regular occurrence. This is good from a financial standpoint because women tend to be more financially secure as they get older and are established in their careers. The bad news however is that our biological clocks don't seem to care about that. They refuse to stand still and as we age our eggs age with us making it harder to conceive.

For a while now, we have been hearing that 35 is the magic cut off point and that a woman's fertility declines at that age dramatically. Now we are hearing that the deterioration of the eggs begin even sooner. Researchers are now saying it begins in the late twenties. Women are born with all the eggs they will ever have. A little girl is born with *all* her eggs and that is a lifetime supply. Women don't make new eggs. This means that women who are serious about babies and career need to make serious decisions so that they can have both of their dreams. It's not that it is impossible to get pregnant after 35. The problem is that it gets harder and sometimes there are issues with the woman's eggs that may cause ailments like Down's syndrome and autism in the child.

The Effects Of Aging On Male Fertility

So far, we have looked at the effects of aging on female

fertility, for centuries it was assumed that when a couple could not conceive it was the woman's fault. We are now discovering that the male partner's fertility plays a pivotal role in conception. We have heard so many stories about men in their fifties, sixties and even seventies impregnating women that we tend to think it is a given that all men can do this. While it is true that men can produce sperm at any age the quality of the sperm starts deteriorating at the age of 35 as well. Three major factors come into play as a man ages, these are listed below:

Lowering of Sperm Count

As mentioned before a man will likely still produce sperm all through his life, but he will produce a lot less as he ages and once he gets to the age of 35, every year his sperm count will decrease.

Testosterone Levels Decrease With Age

Testosterone is extremely important when it comes to

producing sperm, a decrease in a man's testosterone level can mean that he begins to produce less sperm and also begins to lose energy, this can impact his sex drive and his sexual ability.

Sperm Abnormality

As a man ages, his sperm is more likely to produce genetic mutations that can cause abnormalities in a child he produces, no matter what the age of the woman he impregnates. In fact, as a man ages his sperm is more likely to produce a child with Down's syndrome and other forms of retardation, including schizophrenia.

If you are reading this and you are over 35 and want to conceive you might be tempted to become discouraged, do not be, this book is about arming you with the knowledge you need to achieve your dreams of having a child as quickly as possible.

Chapter 2

The Ovulation and Menstrual Cycles

You probably already know a lot about the birds and the bees but a refresher course in how your body prepares itself for pregnancy doesn't hurt. The two cycles discussed in this chapter are closely linked, in fact, they are like a circle, and it is hard to know where one begins and where one ends. We are going to look closely at both of them as they play a key role in pregnancy achievement.

The Ovulation Cycle

Ovulation begins when an egg is released from a woman's ovary, this happens once per menstrual cycle and is also part of the ovulation cycle. The actual time of ovulation can vary greatly from woman to woman. This is because the length of a woman's menstrual cycle can be as little as 24 days to as much as 36 days.

Ovulation mainly happens in the middle of the menstrual cycle but can also occur as early as eight days into the cycle. Knowing when you ovulate is the key to pregnancy achievement.

What you should know about ovulation:

1. An egg lives for twelve to twenty four hours.

2. Only one egg is released during ovulation but sometimes more than one is released, and this can result in fraternal twins.

3. It is not unusual to experience spotting during ovulation.

4. When an egg is released, implantation can take place six or twelve days later.

5. A woman is born with all the eggs she will ever have (already mentioned but bears repeating).

6. Mittelschmerz or middle pain is experienced by some women near the ovaries right before they ovulate.

7. Sometimes women have their periods and ovulation has not taken place, this is called anovulation. Sometimes, it is the opposite, a woman may ovulate but have no period.

The Ovulation cycle is made up of two parts, the first phase is known as the follicular phase and it begins on the first day of your last menstrual period and goes on until the time of ovulation. The second part of the cycle begins after you have ovulated and is known as the luteal phase, it starts from the day you ovulate and ends the first day you notice bleeding which signals the start of your period. This is the time in which a fertilized egg will implant in the uterine wall, so the luteal phase is an important part of the ovulation cycle. The luteal phase usually lasts between twelve to sixteen days. If it lasts under ten days it cannot sustain a pregnancy and medication must be given to correct it. The good news is that this problem is easily treated once it is discovered. As mentioned earlier, understanding when you ovulate is the key to getting pregnant. Having intercourse at least three to five days before or on the day of ovulation increases your chances of having a baby.

The Menstrual Cycle

When a girl reaches puberty she has about twenty thousand eggs and less than fifteen of them will try to reach maturity during each menstrual cycle. Every menstrual cycle your body prepares itself for pregnancy. Follicle stimulating hormone (FSH) sends messages to the eggs in the ovary to start the maturation process. Every single egg is in a follicle of its own. Each of these follicles start producing the hormone estrogen. This hormone goes surging through each of the follicles and the one that gets the biggest, the fastest is the one that finds itself released during ovulation. Large amounts of luteinizing hormones are triggered by the hormone estrogen and that is what actually causes the egg to be released. The other eggs dissolve and fall apart, eventually. Sometimes, the egg is released with such force that some women will feel a sharp pain coming from the ovary where this occurs. The follicle that the egg is enclosed in becomes ruptured and the luteinizing hormones cause the follicle to be transformed into the corpus luteum. The corpus luteum in turn starts secreting estrogen and progesterone which prepares the endometrial lining of the uterus for the fertilized egg. The corpus luteum will stay behind for about twelve to sixteen days. The progesterone that the corpus luteum releases prevents any other egg from being released and creates a barrier. However on rare occasions, an extra egg slips past and this usually produces fraternal twins.

By staying behind, the corpus luteum and the progesterone it is releasing gives the endometrium enough time to become strong enough to sustain the egg if it has been fertilized. Naturally, if the egg is not fertilized then the work done by progesterone on the corpus luteum and the endometrium become unnecessary, so the corpus luteum disintegrates causing less estrogen and progesterone to be released. The endometrial lining then becomes quite weak and it then begins to shed in the form of blood, this shedding is known as menstruation.

Chapter 3

What To Avoid And What To Embrace When Trying To Conceive

There are several things that can destroy your chances of conceiving quickly, below are the top offenders and the top defenders of your fertility.

Do Avoid:

1. Excessive Amounts Of Vitamin C

While the right amount of Vitamin C can help to enhance cervical fluid (this is the vaginal fluid that sperm swim in to get to the egg). Too much (more than 750 mg-100mg) can have the opposite effect, so avoid high dosages of this vitamin.

2. Stress

Stress is the enemy of fertility, when a woman is stressed it can affect when she ovulates. Sometimes, stress prevents ovulation from occurring. If ovulation fails to take place then fertilization and conception cannot occur.

3. Lubricants

Many of the lubricants that couples use when trying to conceive may actually be killing sperm. In order to avoid this, try using egg whites or a sperm friendly lubricant called *Pre-seed*, if you need lubrication.

4. Avoid Certain Types of Fish

Some fish contain mercury and can cause harm when you are trying to conceive, these include, king mackerel, shark, swordfish, tile fish (golden or white snapper), orange roughy, Spanish mackerel, marlin and tuna steaks. Fish is high in Omega-3 fatty acids and protein and is an excellent source of nutrients for those trying to conceive and as long as you avoid the ones with mercury you will be fine.

5. Avoid Caffeine

There have been numerous studies done on this and while

some studies may seem to contradict the conventional wisdom, it is better to be safe than sorry. When it comes to caffeine it is always better to be cautious. So while you are trying to get pregnant, it is best that you avoid drinking too much coffee and try to cut back on caffeinated beverages.

6. Avoid Alcohol

Alcohol will severely diminish your fertility, if you drink it excessively and it is not just a problem for women. It reduces testosterone levels in men, as well as sperm count.

7. Avoid Smoking

Cigarettes are not only damaging to your lungs but they also put your fertility at risk. When you smoke a cigarette, as many as 7000 chemicals pass through your body, is it any wonder why it can cause ovulation problems, miscarriage in women, low sperm count as well as erectile dysfunction in men. There is a 23% decrease in sperm concentration for men who smoke, concentration refers to the amount of sperm produced. There is also a 13% decrease in the motility of the sperm among men who smoke, this means there is a 13% decrease in their sperm's ability to swim to the egg in order to fertilize it.

8. Avoid Heat

Most men know that saunas, hot tubs and tight underwear are bad for their fertility because heat damages sperm. What they may not know is that studies have now found that men may now be endangering their fertility with their laptops. The heat generated from a laptop has now been linked to infertility in some men. Men should place their laptops on tables when using them and avoid putting them in their laps.

Do :

1. Take Folic Acid

New studies have shown that both partners should take folic acid as this reduces the chance of birth defects such as spina bifida. Previously, this supplement was highly encouraged for women only, 400 mcg is a good dosage although some people take it in higher amounts. It is a water soluble vitamin so the excess is passed out in the urine.

2. Get A Check Up

A full checkup should be done before you and your partner decide to conceive, in order to be sure that you are both healthy and fit.

3. Eat Fertility Superfoods:

-broccoli

Broccoli is high in folic acid which prevents spina bifida in the fetus and also in Vitamin c which assists in ovulation.

-cabbage

Cabbage has a nutrient known as Di-Indole Methane, this

helps to prevent fibroids and greatly decreases the chances of a woman developing endometriosis..

-yams

Yams help the body to produce more estrogen, this assists with ovulation.

-eggs

Egg yolk is rich in choline, it helps in the prevention of spina bifida.

-sprouts

Sprouts help to make cervical fluid (fluid used by sperm to swim to the egg) less acidic. Acidic cervical fluid kills sperm.

-avocados

Avocados contain Vitamin E, this increases the ability of sperm to swim to the egg.

-Olive oil

Olive oil contains unsaturated fats these help to prevent ovulation problems.

-garlic

Contains selenium which is an anti-oxidant that prevents miscarriage.

4. Try lovemaking more than baby making

-Enjoy sexual intercourse with your partner, this relieves stress which aids in conception, it is tempting when you are desperate to conceive to forget about enjoying sex and turn it into a project, in the long run this does more harm than good.

Chapter 4

Sexual Positions That Help You To Get Pregnant

Some experts argue that any sexual position can make a woman pregnant, while little can be said to contest this fact, it is worth noting that no one can argue that the closer semen is deposited to the cervix the better the chances of conceiving.

Let's examine some of the best positions for getting sperm as close to the cervix as possible:

Missionary Style:

The missionary position is well known, this is when the male is on top of the female. It is one of the best positions for conception.

The Missionary Style With Butt Lift:

The missionary style with the butt lift involves the

missionary position with one variation, the man lifts the woman's entire lower body towards him before he ejaculates. This gets sperm very close to the cervix.

Flipped Missionary

In this position the woman lies flat on her tummy with a pillow under her hips for elevation to allow for deep penetration.

Rear Entry

This position is good for any woman trying to conceive, but if you have a tipped uterus then this position is perfect for you. It allows the man to have greater control, so he can penetrate deeply.

Take A Rest

Laying down for fifteen minutes after intercourse may actually help! Researchers in Amsterdam discovered in 2009, that women who lay down for fifteen minutes after artificial insemination were 50% more likely to conceive. There's no reason this shouldn't work after intercourse as well.

Chapter 5

Fertility Signs

There are two kinds of fertility signs, they are known as primary and secondary fertility signs. Primary signs are those signs that are definitive. They are your body's clues that tell you that ovulation is on the way and they are 100% reliable, if you know how to correctly analyze them. Secondary fertility signs are those signs that are used as a backup for the primary signs, in other words, secondary signs help to confirm the primary signs.

Primary Fertility Signs

The primary fertility signs are:

Your waking or basal body temperature

Your waking or basal temperature will tell you over the course of about three or four months, whether or not you ovulate. Your temperature will often be lower before you ovulate and then make a sharp rise after you have ovulated. Some women experience a sharp dip in temperature around the time of ovulation and then a dramatic rise after ovulation.

Cervical Fluid

Cervical Fluid or mucus is that fluid that a woman secretes naturally from her cervix, it flows down to the vagina. The type of cervical fluid a woman is producing is directly related to where she is in her cycle. Throughout the cycle, cervical fluid goes from moist to lotiony or creamy and finally to egg white consistency. A woman is most fertile when she is producing egg white cervical fluid. Learning how to identify this fertility sign will tell a woman when she is fertile and when she is infertile during her menstrual cycle.

Cervical Position

Every month your cervix changes position depending on

whether you are fertile or not. The cervix is usually firm, low and closed but as ovulation approaches it becomes soft, high, open and very wet from the cervical fluid it pushes out.

Secondary Fertility Signs

Secondary fertility signs are not experienced by all women, but for those who are lucky enough to have them they provide extra clues as to what is happening inside their bodies during any given cycle. Here are a few common secondary fertility signs:

1. Pain or aching near ovaries
2. Water retention
3. Breast tenderness
4. Abdominal bloating
5. Some women experience a sharp pain in the ovary from which the egg is released.
6. Some women may notice that one side of their

vulva (vaginal lips) swells. This usually occurs on the side where the ovary that released the egg is located

7. Increased need for sexual intercourse

Chapter 6

The Natural Way To Find Out If You Ovulate

Your waking or basal body temperature

Your waking or basal temperature will tell you over the course of about three or four months, whether or not you ovulate.

Taking Your Temperature

Temperature taking is done using a basal thermometer. A basal thermometer is different from other thermometers, in that, it measures the lowest temperatures. You should take your temperature orally every morning at about the same time, after at least three to four hours of sleep. Use a digital basal thermometer, since they usually beep to tell you that the temperature is taken. You may also take your temperature vaginally. Whether you take your temperature orally or vaginally, you must use the same method every time you take your temperature.

Important Points

1. Take your temperature as soon as you wake up. It is best to keep the thermometer by your bed for easy access.

2. A severe rise in temperature usually indicates that ovulation has taken place. Some women see a severe dip then a sharp rise.

3. A sharp dip in temperature usually indicates the day of ovulation.

4. Illness can throw off your temperature reading.

5. Sleeping later than you normally would, throws off your temperature. Your temperature may rise 1/10 of a degree for every half an hour of extra sleep.

Benefits of temperature taking and charting

1. Over a period of three or four months you'll definitely find out whether or not you ovulating.

2. You'll know when your period is near.

3. You'll find out if you have a long enough "luteal phase" to sustain an implanted egg.

4. You will be able to pinpoint pregnancy before taking a test.

Charting Your Temperature

Temperatures must be recorded on a basal chart. Getting a basal temperature chart is pretty easy, simply do a google search and download and print one for free, in either Celsius or Fahrenheit. It is best to start taking your temperature as soon as your period ends, so that you can record a full cycle. Use a blue ink pen or black ink pen to connect the dots, every morning after you take your waking temperature with a basal thermometer. Here are some examples with explanation.

Ann's Chart

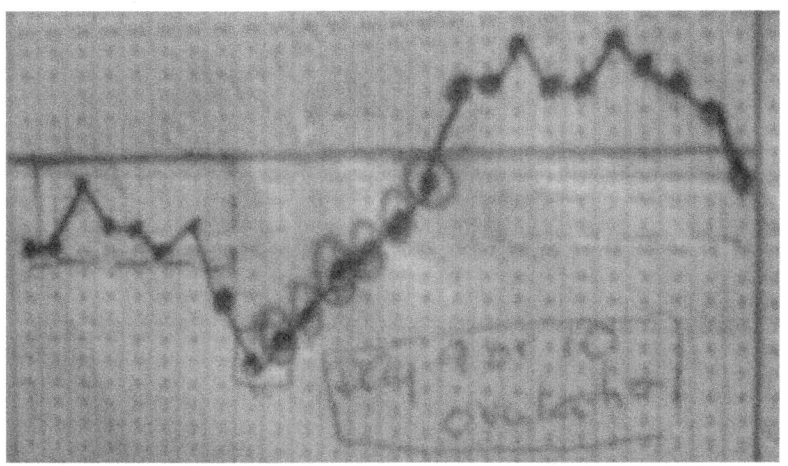

If you count from the first dot, you will notice that the lowest dip in temperature occurs on day 9, clearly showing ovulation (Ann was unsure if ovulation happened on day 9 or 10). It is highly unlikely that it was day 10 since the temperature started rising at this time and continued its upward trend. Notice the horizontal line running across the page, this is the coverline. The coverline helps to identify when the non-fertile days begin and the length of the luteal phase.

Start counting from the beginning of the chart to day 16. Notice that the first six days of temperature rise before the final dramatic rise in temperature on day 16 are circled in order to assist with the drawing of the coverline. The coverline should always be drawn above the highest temperature of these six days. The luteal phase or infertile part of Ann's cycle began on day 10, immediately after ovulation. If you count from day 10 onwards, you will see that her luteal phase is 16 days long.

Take a look at the drop in temperature towards the end of the cycle as menstruation approaches again, this signals a drop in estrogen levels.

DRAWING A COVERLINE

1. First find a temperature on your chart that shows a temperature rise of .2 degrees or more.

2. Draw circles around the previous six days before this dramatic rise in temperature.

3. Find the highest of the six circled temperatures (the highest of the six may be the 2nd, 3rd, 4th, 5th or 6th temperature). It doesn't matter. In Ann's case it was the 6th temperature that was the highest.

4. Draw a straight line that is one-tenth /0.1 of a degree higher than that of the highest of the circled temperatures. This line is the coverline, the coverline runs horizontally across your chart.

Another of Ann's Charts

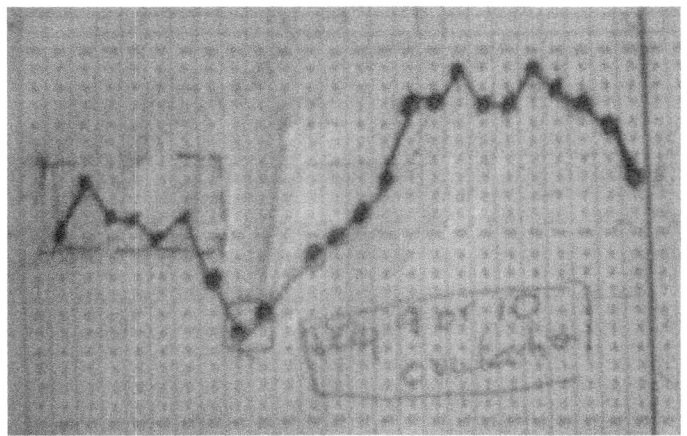

Here Ann begins charting on the second day after her period is completed. You can see a sharp temperature dip on day 9, indicating ovulation. Ann is unsure and notes that it might be day 10. This is erroneous because even though she missed charting on day 11, from day 12 onward we see a continuation of the rise in temperature that began on day 10, this shows that ovulation did in fact take place on day 9. The temperature makes a dramatic rise on day 16. The coverline is missing here, but it should be drawn one tenth of a degree above the dot at day 15 which shows the highest temperature of the previous six days before the dramatic rise that occurs on day 16. Notice that she has drawn a vertical line where the chart ends. This is the correct way to indicate the end of the cycle.

Counting from day 10, we can see that her luteal phase is 16 days long. This means that she can support a pregnancy. Luteal phases that are less than 10 days will not sustain a pregnancy. The luteal phase and its role in sustaining pregnancy or causing miscarriages, as well as treatment for short luteal phases will be discussed in Chapter 10.

Note

If you have high temperatures for more than 18 days after ovulation this indicates pregnancy.

Ovulation Predictor Kits

If you find that checking your waking temperature is a bit too tedious you can use an ovulation predictor kit to try and pinpoint whether or not you are ovulating.

Ovulation Predictor Kits (OPK) work by analyzing the

amount of (LH) luteinizing hormone in the urine. The tricky part is that LH may rise without ovulation taking place. That is why ovulation predictor kits can be unreliable when it comes to understanding the ovulation cycle and when you ovulate.

Additionally, sometimes a woman may have two LH surges making it difficult to know which one is the real surge, when this happens a woman who is trying to conceive may incorrectly time sex and end up not conceiving because the egg was actually released during the second surge.

The kit does not give any information about the status of the cervical fluid which is the key to detecting impending ovulation which increases the chances of conception. In fact, most of the time when OPK's show a surge in LH, cervical fluid has started to dry up and without fertile quality cervical fluid the vagina's environment becomes hostile to sperm, and this decreases the chances of conception.

The best way to actually tell when you are ovulating is to get to know your body and watch for the signs that you are ovulating by checking cervical fluid yourself, as your body provides you with plenty of accurate clues once you know what to look for. In the next chapter we will look at how to use cervical fluid to pinpoint ovulation.

Chapter 7

Find Out Exactly When You Ovulate

Identifying exactly when you ovulate is the key to having a baby. The best way to know when you are about to ovulate is not by reading your waking/basal temperature chart and looking for temperature shifts. It is also not by using an Ovulation Predictor Kit (OPK). The best way, is to learn how to observe your cervical fluid so that you can identify when you are most fertile.

Women are actually fertile for about six or seven days. This is because a man's sperm is able to survive for up to five days and can fertilize an egg released within that period. A woman is also fertile on the day she ovulates, some experts add an extra day, just in case one or more egg has been released, this is a rare event and can result in fraternal twins if both eggs are fertilized.

Knowing the breakdown of the fertile window can help you to better understand how to conceive a child.

Here is the breakdown:

5 days (sperm survival) +the day you ovulate+ one extra day just in case an extra egg was released= 7 days

If you are trying to conceive it is always better to try within the first 6 days of the fertile window, since this is the time of high fertility. In order not to miss your fertile window you must have some idea when you ovulate, in order to do this, the best thing to do is to start tracking your cervical fluid as soon as your period ends. Cervical fluid often starts off sticky or pasty then becomes lotiony or milky and finally it gets an egg white consistency. Egg white consistency tells you that you are about to ovulate. This helps you to have the best chance at conceiving.

Watching your cervical fluid is a natural ovulation calculator and is an extremely effective way of predicting ovulation and tracking your Ovulation cycle. If you are serious about conception then you should never miss an opportunity to have intercourse whenever you observe lotiony or milky fluid, although egg white cervical fluid is the most fertile.

Let us look at exactly how you should go about checking your cervical fluid:

Observing Cervical Fluid

Start observing your cervical fluid immediately after your period. You can observe cervical fluid whenever you go to the bathroom. Separate your vaginal lips and use clean fingers or tissue to remove and observe the fluid coming from the entrance of the vagina.

--Check your underwear. The seat of your underwear often provides clues to the type of cervical fluid your cervix is excreting.

--Take a peak after a bowel movement, often egg white cervical fluid is clearly visible, as it hangs out of the vagina. Look in the toilet water too, egg white cervical fluid will form itself into a ball in the water.

--If you can't detect the fluid externally, use your index and middle finger to gently pull fluid from the cervix itself.

Even when the observation of cervical fluid is done right and intercourse is perfectly timed, bear in mind that there is still only a 25% chance of conception every cycle. Some couples are lucky and conceive right away. Some need three months, some need six months and some need a year. In general, if you and your partner are healthy then it should happen within a year. If not, then it is definitely time to see a doctor to check for fertility issues, especially if the woman is over 35.

Cervical Position

Cervical Position is a fertility sign you can use to back up cervical fluid checks. It is not hard to check but it is not for everyone, if the thought of touching your cervix is a little scary in the beginning, know that this feeling is completely normal. This step is optional and is mainly for women who find all the primary fertility signs confusing and for those who may want to pull cervical fluid off the cervix itself.

Checking Your Cervix

1. TRIM YOUR NAILS.
2. Wash your hands thoroughly.
3. The best time to check is usually when you shower or take a bath.
4. Squat or stand and raise one leg on your tub or a footrest of your choice. Squatting is also acceptable, whichever position you choose, make sure you use the same position every time you check, so that

your cervix is always the same height.

5. Use your middle finger.
6. Check if the cervix is firm, soft or a texture in between.
7. Check if it is low, high or just about halfway.
8. Check if it is closed, open or partially open.
9. Check if you feel any cervical fluid (sticky, lotiony, eggwhite) or dry.
10. You can pull cervical fluid off your cervix using your *middle* and *index finger*.

Note

As you approach ovulation your cervix becomes open, soft and it also rises.

Chapter 8

Selecting Your Baby's Gender

It is not uncommon for parents to want to select the gender of their child. This chapter is thrown in as a bonus for those who may be interested in trying these methods. Obviously, if you are struggling to conceive then the gender of the child may be the last thing on your mind. However, there are others who might feel differently. This chapter is provided to help them realize their dreams of having a little boy or girl.

The easiest and least invasive method of trying to select the gender of your child is the Shettles method. The Shettles method is named after the doctor who created it.

Dr. Shettles claims a 75 % to 90 % success rate using this method. To date this is the best method that can be used at home to enhance a couples chances of conceiving a boy or a girl. Shettles theorized that there are two types of sperm, one which carries the X chromosome and one which carries Y chromosome. Y sperm are those sperm that produce males, he found that they had a small round head and were the fastest swimmers but that they lived for a short period of time. The X sperm was the female sperm, they had larger oval heads and they moved much slower than Y sperm but they were stronger and able to survive for a longer period.

Given the perfect set of circumstances for conception which usually means that a woman is secreting egg-white quality cervical fluid and is just about to ovulate. The Y sperm containing male chromosomes have the best chance of fertilizing the egg if the woman has intercourse as close to ovulation as possible, this is because the X or "female" sperm will find it difficult to out swim them. The rich cervical fluid allows the Y sperm to swim fast and get to the egg quickly and create a boy. The opposite is the case when trying to conceive a girl, instead of having sex close to ovulation you should have intercourse further away from ovulation, ideally three or four days before so that only the slower X sperm that also live longer are able to survive.

This is the crux of the Shettles method. If you study this method you will see that you must be aware of when you ovulate, it is also worth learning how to monitor cervical fluid, as discussed in the previous chapter as this will assist you in identifying how far or how close you are to ovulation.

Chapter 9

Am I Pregnant?

Now that you know how to maximize your chances of getting pregnant, let us look at some of the common signs of pregnancy.

Pregnancy Symptoms

- **Constant urination**- When your uterus expands it tends to push against the bladder causing you to urinate frequently.

- **Breast tenderness**- Caused by excessive amounts of the hormone estrogen and progesterone, which is preparing your breasts to feed your baby.

- **Tiredness**- As the hormone progesterone races through the body tiredness and fatigue begins to set in.

- **Implantation spotting** -Pinkish brown discharge that occurs when an egg is fertilized by a sperm and it implants in the uterine wall, this often occurs 8-12 days after ovulation, may be accompanied by implantation cramping.

- **Implantation cramping** - Pain that often feels like menstrual cramps, this happens when the fertilized egg implants in the uterus and may be accompanied by implantation bleeding.

- **Nausea and vomiting-** This is another common feature of pregnancy and it is caused by high hormone levels, heightened sensitivity to odors and the fact that some women have sensitive stomachs that react to the changes in pregnancy.

-**Excessive hunger and food aversions** –You may find yourself getting hungry quicker and suddenly disliking foods you once enjoyed.

-**Abdominal bloating**-Progesterone relaxes the stomach muscles, slowing down digestion, so that nutrients can get to your baby, unfortunately this can cause bloating, gas and flatulence.

Let's take a closer look at two major indicators of pregnancy that you may notice before you do a pregnancy test. These signs do not happen to everyone so do not be alarmed if they do not happen to you.

Implantation Bleeding Or Spotting

Implantation bleeding or spotting occurs in some women about six to twelve days after conception. This bleeding occurs when the egg implants into the endometrial lining of the uterus. This may cause a bit of blood to shed. This bleeding or spotting is either dark brown or pinkish in appearance. It usually lasts for about two days, although it can go on for longer in some cases. If you notice this for about a week, consult your doctor. Implantation bleeding normally occurs about a week or a few days before your period would normally occur. It occurs in about 25% of pregnant women.

Note

Blood pregnancy tests usually give a positive reading about 3-4 days after implantation has occurred and in 4-5 days with urine tests.

Implantation Cramping

Some women experience cramping when the egg implants in the lining of the uterus. These cramps are often similar to menstrual cramps. Cramping usually occurs along with implantation bleeding or spotting, but it may also occur on its own.

Pregnancy Quiz

Wondering if you are pregnant? Take this pregnancy quiz and find out, simply answer yes or no. Keep count of how many times you say yes!

1. Is your period more than one week late?
2. Are your breasts unusually sore?

3. Are your areola (area around your nipple) getting darker?

4. Are you feeling nauseous and have an upset stomach that lasts all day or for several hours?

5. Are you starting to go to the bathroom to urinate more frequently?

6. Have you experienced implantation spotting?

7. Are you feeling more tired and need to take a nap more often than usual?

8. Are you experiencing pain in your lower back or headaches in the morning?

9. Do you chart your basal temperature, if so has your temperature remained high for 18 consecutive days?

If you answered yes to number 1 and 5 other questions in the pregnancy quiz then it is time to take a pregnancy test.

Pregnancy Tests

Urine Pregnancy Tests should be done after a missed period, this will ensure that there is a high enough human chorionic gonadotrophin (hCG) level in the urine for detection.

If you observe implantation bleeding or spotting then you should wait at least 4-5 days, as previously mentioned, to get accurate results. It is best to use the first urine of the morning as this usually has the highest concentration of the hCG hormone.

Urine pregnancy tests done at home should in no way replace a blood test done by your doctor.

Chapter 10

When Pregnancy Goes Wrong

Causes of Miscarriages

Miscarriage is a term used when a pregnancy is aborted naturally. They usually take place in the first three months of a pregnancy and about one in five pregnancies will end in miscarriage. Naturally, if the pregnancy was wanted this creates emotional disturbance, as a woman and her partner come to terms with the loss, sometimes professional help may be necessary to cope with the grief. For some women the recovery happens quickly, for others it takes more time.

Women may suffer from recurrent miscarriages without actually knowing it because these miscarriage happens very early in the pregnancy. This is one reason why in depth knowledge of your fertility is so important.

The most serious and dangerous infections that cause

miscarriages are malaria, chlamydia, listeria and infections in a man's sperm. The herpes virus is also considered dangerous in pregnancy as well, especially if a woman has an outbreak in the first five months of pregnancy, this virus may cause a miscarriage. Viruses such as German measles, mumps and hepatitis A and B are also dangerous viruses which may lead to a miscarriage.

Miscarriages can also be caused by problems with the uterus, some women may have a weak cervix and if this is the case, it may begin to break apart while the fetus is not fully grown, this will result in a miscarriage. The term used to describe this is "incompetent cervix".

The shape of a woman's cervix affects its ability to allow the fetus to grow or stay in the uterus. In such cases the woman's doctor is likely to stitch the womb to prevent the cervix from completely dilating.

Women are now taking longer to have babies and unfortunately age does play a huge part in whether or not a woman is able to carry a pregnancy to term, since age affects the viability of the fertilized egg. However, the most common cause of miscarriage tends to be chromosomal irregularities, which result in the pregnancy being naturally terminated.

Symptoms of A Miscarriage

Bleeding is one sure sign that a miscarriage is likely to occur. The bleeding is usually bright red in color. Once bleeding starts to occur, it means a miscarriage is threatened, it doesn't necessarily mean that the pregnancy is lost. Many women experience this kind of early bleeding and go on to have a healthy baby, some women bleed throughout their entire pregnancy and still carry healthy babies to term. It is when cramping occurs along with the heavy bleeding and clots start being passed, that it becomes clear that the pregnancy is being terminated. Still there are a few exceptions to this, a small percentage of women have reported bleeding and seeing clots and still carrying the pregnancy to term.

Nausea, vomiting and fatigue are common symptoms during pregnancy but these symptoms are also signs of a miscarriage as well.

Miscarriages are devastating but they do answer some very important fertility questions with positive answers. They prove that a woman is in fact ovulating, this is extremely important because there can be no pregnancy if an egg is not released for fertilization. They also prove that the fallopian tubes are not blocked and that the woman produces enough high quality cervical mucus or fluid to assist sperm in swimming towards the egg. Finally, they prove that the male partner's sperm count is sufficient.

Luteal Phase

In Chapter 6 the luteal phase was discussed and you learned how to identify it on your chart. The luteal phase is the part of the woman's cycle between ovulation and menstruation. However, if the luteal phase is under 10 days, the egg may not get a chance to implant and a miscarriage may result. A luteal phase shorter than 10 days is considered a luteal defect.

Treatment for Luteal Defect

50-100mg of B6 Vitamin, throughout the month can lengthen the luteal phase. Vitamin B6 is water-soluble and can be taken in higher doses, but it is rarely needed in dosages above 100mg for a luteal defect.

Progesterone cream may also be rubbed into the skin of the neck, arm or chest over the course of several days. About half a teaspoon twice daily is usually adequate.

You may also consult your doctor who will usually prescribe a drug call Clomid.

Ectopic Pregnancy

Sometimes a pregnancy implants outside the uterus. This usually occurs in the fallopian tube. The fallopian tube cannot sustain a growing embryo, because of this it hemorrhages and rupture occurs. Women with ectopic pregnancies often have bleeding and lower abdominal pain.

Treatment For Ectopic Pregnancy

Part or all of the fallopian tube may be surgically removed. Smaller ectopic pregnancies are easier to deal with, the woman is usually injected with a drug called methotrexate and this causes the cells to die, slowly terminating the ectopic pregnancy.

Chapter 11

Major Causes Of Female Infertility

Anovulation

Anovulation occurs when ovulation doesn't take place, this means that throughout the course of a menstrual cycle no egg has been released. Anovulation is generally the reason for a missed period. Since the most blatant sign of anovulation is a missed menstruation and this is also a primary sign or pregnancy, a lot of women who have this condition erroneously think they are expecting.

Unfortunately, anovulation is an extremely frequent occurrence in women with fertility issues. If a woman doesn't ovulate, she definitely will not get pregnant, since ovulation is the key to getting pregnant. When anovulation is detected via missed menstruation, then a woman will be more likely to seek treatment. However, there are cases where bleeding takes place without ovulation occurring and this can cause anovulation to go on for a long time before a woman becomes aware of it. It should be noted that this kind of bleeding is somewhat distinct in color and shade and the quantity not as heavy as typical menstruation, which is a signal that something is not right. Additionally, in a number of instances, the bleeding is pain-free and irregular, nonetheless, many women still mistakenly believe they are having a period.

Anovulation may have several triggers, these include, anxiety, some varieties of medications, nervousness, imbalances with hormones, strenuous workout or excessive weight gain as well as excessive weight loss. Once you find out you're not ovulating you should verify this with your physician as soon as possible and discover what exactly has brought about this problem. Based on what is discovered, your doctor will decide on the necessary treatment. Thankfully, there are numerous treatment options now available for anovulation and it is not a problem that will forever stamp the pain of infertility on a woman.

Clomifene citrate (or clomid) is the medication that is often used to deal with anovulation. Clomid blocks estrogen receptors in the hypothalamus of the brain. The hypothalamus is then stimulated to produce follicle stimulating hormones (FSH) and luteinizing hormones (LH). These hormones stimulate the ovaries and allow ovulation to take place. In addition, clomid has a positive impact on the production of cervical fluid, because it causes it to have an egg white quality that makes it easier for sperm to survive and swim in order to fertilize an egg.

Polycystic Ovary Syndrome

A woman may suffer from polycystic ovary syndrome (PCOS) when cysts develop in the ovaries. The ovaries will then produce more testosterone than is required and ovulation will become erratic and may not occur every month. Some women may not menstruate, because the follicles in the ovaries do not develop.

There are many factors that are believed to cause Polycystic Ovary Syndrome, a few of them are insulin deficiency, heredity and obesity. Insulin is a hormone that is made in the pancreas and it is used by the body to control blood sugar levels. Women who have PCOS often develop a resistance to insulin. This resistance causes the body to produce more insulin along with the hormone testosterone. This interferes with the follicular development in the ovary which hinders ovulation and menstruation. The compounded effect is the inability to conceive or problems conceiving. Excessive amounts of testosterone often produce an overgrowth of hair on the body, including facial hair in some cases. The increase in insulin may also cause weight gain. Being even slightly overweight can cause the condition to worsen, since excess weight may increase resistance to insulin forcing an increase in insulin production.

The major symptoms of Polycystic Ovarian Syndrome are as follows:

1. Women with PCOS have irregular periods or they may not have any period of all. At least 70 percent of women with PCOS have menstruation problems.
2. Women with PCOS do not ovulate, or ovulate infrequently.
3. Some have facial, chest and abdominal hair.
4. Acne may be present well past puberty.
5. Thinning of the hair may occur, balding often resembles male pattern baldness.

There are varied treatments for this condition, these include lifestyle and diet changes if the woman is obese. Hormones may be given through the use of birth control pills that contain the hormone progesterone. Diabetes medication which slows down the production of insulin may also be used in addition to fertility drugs such as Clomid.

Endometriosis

Endometrial cells are shed each month during menstruation. Endometriosis occurs when there is an overgrowth of endometrial cells. The overgrowths mimic the endometrial cells that are found inside the uterus and they may attach themselves to tissues surrounding the womb. Endometriosis implants are often found on the fallopian tubes, ovaries, on the surface of the pelvic cavity, cervix or vagina. These implants are never cancerous.

Endometriosis often affects women who are still in their reproductive years. When it affects these women it makes fertility a challenge or it may stop the possibility of reproduction altogether. Most women who have endometriosis are between the ages of 25 to 35. Although, girls as young as 11 have been known to develop endometriosis. Many women who have endometriosis have no symptoms of the condition. However, some have severe pelvic pain. Endometriosis is one of the main causes of hysterectomies. It also seems there is some ethnic bias where endometriosis in concerned, as it is a condition more common to Caucasian women, than Asian women or women of African descent.

The reason that endometriosis occurs has been the cause of much speculation between doctors and scientists. Some scientists believe that the areas that line the pelvic cavity contain cells that are able to grow and form into other tissues. Other scientists hypothesize that endometrial tissue gets into different places in the body when menstrual flow goes back into the fallopian tubes, as well as the pelvic cavity during a woman's period.

Progestins are often used for treating endometriosis.

Gonadotropin-releasing hormone analogs or oral contraceptives may also be used. The Gonadotropin-releasing hormone analogs (GnRH analogs) are used to relieve pain. They work by significantly slowing the production of estrogen in the ovaries and by curbing the release of hormones from the pituitary gland. This causes a kind of menopause and the woman's menstrual period will stop. Progestins are very powerful and are prescribed for women whose pain does not subside with the use of GnRH analogs or oral contraceptives.

Fibroids

 Many women get fibroids, however, it is largely dependent on age. The older you get the more likely you are to have them. Women who have never been pregnant are at a higher risk. Smoking, obesity, being of African descent (women of African descent get fibroids at least three times as often as women of European or Asian descent) puts a woman at higher risk for fibroids.

Fibroids are tumors that are benign and they rarely become malignant. The impact of fibroids on fertility is dependent on the location of the fibroid. Fibroids can be submucosal, meaning they are under the lining of the uterine cavity or they can be intramural, this means that they are located in the muscle of the uterus. When they are very near to the outside of a woman's uterus they are considered subserosal.

Polypoid fibroids are located on stalks inside the uterus and pedunculated fibroids are on the outside of the uterus. A woman can have a single fibroid or she may have multiple fibroids, some of them may be big and some of them may be small. Fibroids that are in the lining of the uterine cavity seem to pose the most danger to fertility and the ones located in the muscles of the uterus sometimes cause fertility issues, the effect is dependent on their size. Many women who have fibroids get pregnant and deliver safely. Fibroids have only been found to be the sole cause of infertility in 2% of cases where a woman cannot conceive.

Symptoms that you may have fibroids include, heavy periods, bladder problems, pelvic discomfort and pain, lower back pain and pain during sexual intercourse, these symptoms vary and are largely dependent on the size and location of the fibroid.

Surgical removal of fibroids involve going through the cervix using a hysteroscope to remove fibroids that are under the lining of the cavity. Removal of these types of fibroids will usually result in successful attempts at pregnancy if they had been involved in infertility. The procedure to remove them is called a hysteroscopic myomectomy. If other types of fibroids are removed they generally do not increase the success rate of pregnancy and are likely to leave scar tissue that will further hinder a woman's chance at conception.

Uterine artery embolization is often used as an alternative to surgery, as well as magnetic resonance focused ultrasound. However, studies have shown that there are increased risk for miscarriages as well as post-partum hemorrhage and greater risk for cesarean deliveries with these treatments.

Alcohol and Pregnancy

Women who are attempting to conceive should reduce alcohol consumption or stay away from alcohol altogether. If you are trying to conceive a child then it is best that you do not consume more than 175 milliliters of alcohol per week. Alcohol must be avoided throughout pregnancy, but it should especially be avoided in the first trimester when the baby is developing all its vital organs. Alcohol is not pregnancy friendly and if a woman usually drinks she needs to stop immediately, once she discovers she is pregnant.

Alcohol is not only bad for expectant mothers, it also makes getting pregnant harder. Studies show that it can make a woman much less fertile. A study done in Denmark found that drinking anywhere from 1 and 5 drinks per week can decrease a woman's ability to conceive dramatically and having ten drinks or more is even more detrimental to conception. A study carried out at Harvard University focused on couples who were having IVF treatments. The study found that when women drank 525 milliliters or more of alcohol per week they had a 18% less chance of conceiving, while males had a 14% less chance.

High amounts of alcohol significantly lowers testosterone, sperm count and sperm motility. However, the good news is that the effects of alcohol on fertility are reversible, quitting alcohol while you are trying to conceive is always the best option, but if you can't do this it is best to just consume a pint of alcohol per week for men and about a half pint per week for women.

Remember that drinking whether socially or otherwise should always be done in moderation even when a couple is not trying to conceive. As excessive amounts of alcohol do not bode well for a healthy lifestyle in general and should be avoided. Also be sure that you are eating well and exercising since this helps to boost fertility and prevent other health problems. It is best to curb the consumption of alcohol especially if you are undergoing IVF treatments, since alcohol diminishes the effects of these treatments.

Chapter 12

Major Causes Of Male Infertility

Male Infertility

Infertility is largely discussed as being a female problem, unfortunately this is a fallacy which needs to be addressed. While about half of the problems with fertility that couples have are because of fertility issues in the woman, the other forty percent of fertility issues come from problems with the male partner's fertility. The additional ten percent occurs when both the man and the woman have fertility issues. So, it is clearly not a female problem. In centuries past women were stigmatized and criticized harshly when they couldn't have any children, during this time it really never occurred to anyone that her male partner could be the one with fertility issues. This stigma and perception continues today, even in the age of modern medicine.

Testing for fertility in men is not difficult and usually

requires a semen sample. A semen evaluation will figure out if a man is experiencing fertility issues. The semen analysis will try to find out four things about the sperm, these are, its volume, concentration, morphology and motility.

What is volume?

Semen not only consists of sperm, it also contains enzymes and amino acids. When a man has a small amount of ejaculate, it may be that he doesn't secrete enough of these enzymes and amino acids that help to increase sperm volume.

What is concentration?

This is what individuals generally refer to as "sperm count." A small amount of sperm indicates that there are issues with the testicles and hormones may be present that are preventing the man's testicles from creating enough sperm.

What is motility?

The motion of sperm is extremely important to male fertility. If sperm cannot swim properly, it could impact the sperm's capability to get through the cervix and fertilize the egg.

What is morphology?

This speaks to the shape of the sperm. The head of each sperm must have the correct shape in order to bore its way into the egg. If the sperm's head is deformed in any way this will impact its ability to penetrate the egg.

As you can see, there is a lot that can be found out from one sample of semen. If the semen sample turns out to be subfertile then the man's doctor will want to do at least two more analyses, this is for the purpose of comparison. These will be done over a period of two to four weeks in order to confirm the results of the first test.

Varicoceles

Whenever a man experiences diminished sperm count, it is often caused by varicoceles in the scrotal sac. Varicoceles are caused by an enlargement of the veins that are found in the bag of skin that holds the testicles. This bag of skin is called the scrotum, as much as 40% of all men who are infertile suffer from this condition. Sometimes, a man may have this condition and not have infertility issues. The good news is that surgery can improve sperm count by as much as 80%.

Hormonal Deficiency

Another cause of male infertility is hormone deficiency. Insufficient amounts of follicle stimulating hormones (FSH) as well as luteinizing hormones (LH) can cause sperm production to slow down. This hormonal problem is often treated with gonadotropins.

Damaged Sperm Ducts

Sperm ducts can become damaged when a man contracts a sexually transmitted disease. This causes infertility in about 15% of men. Some STD's cause scaring in the vas deferens, effectively preventing sperm from going through the urethra. A varicocele may also be blocking the vas deferens. Sometimes, this condition can be corrected without surgery but often surgery will have to be performed to remove blockage or scarring. This is often effective and resolves the issue immediately.

Testicular Failure

If the amount of reproductive hormones being released by the testicles is insufficient then the result will be testicular failure. This condition can be caused by mumps, tumors,

STD's and drugs. If no sperm is present then there is little that can be done. If sperm is present then fertility drugs can be utilized to increase the number of the sperm.

Sperm Agglutination

This occurs when the man's sperm clumps together, and are not swimming freely. It is caused by the presence of sperm antibodies, these antibodies stick together. About 7% of male infertility is caused by this condition, treatment is fairly simple and usually involves taking Vitamin E and Vitamin C.

Chapter 13

Infertility Testing

At Home Testing

Fertility issues are hard for any woman to deal with, but before you go ahead and get invasive tests, there are a few tests you can do at home to check your fertility.

FSH Strips

A follicle stimulating hormone (FSH) test measures the level of follicle stimulating hormone in the body. By measuring FSH, the test assesses whether or not a woman is producing large amounts of the hormone. Large amounts of FSH mean that egg supply or egg quality is low. This test can be done on the third day of a woman's cycle using FSH strips.

The OV Watch

An OV watch test interprets the amount of sodium chloride ions released by the skin throughout a woman's menstrual cycle. The amount of sodium chloride ions released by the skin fluctuates. Six days before a woman ovulates there is a surge in ions and the watch will spot it.

The OV watch is easy to use, because all you have to do is wear it around the wrist. Most of the times the watch will pinpoint four days when you are fertile before ovulation and one day when you may be fertile after ovulation.

The test that are outlined below are more invasive. These tests are often done by doctors when they believe that something is wrong with a woman's reproductive organs.

Endometrial Biopsy

An endometrial biopsy is done when a piece of the endometrial tissue is removed after twenty one days has passed in the menstrual cycle. An analysis of the tissue is done, to examine how the endometrium developed. The test is done to see if a woman produces a thick enough endometrial lining to facilitate implantation.

Abdominal Ultrasound

Ultrasounds may done abdominally or transvaginally. In the abdominal ultrasound, sound waves bounce off the body and produce an image of the pelvis. When the ultrasound is done transvaginally a better quality image is produced, it is possible to see the development of follicles, fibroids or ovarian cysts which may be hindering fertility.

Sonohystogram

Your doctor may also choose to do a sonohystogram in this procedure a woman's womb is filled with water and saline solution, so that a very clear image of the uterus is produced.

Laparoscopy

A laparoscopy uses a lighted tube which is inserted through a small hole that is made under a woman's navel to view the reproductive system. It helps to find blockages, scar tissues and even endometriosis.

Hysteroscopy

A hysteroscopy uses a small telescope to view the uterus. The telescope is inserted vaginally, this test give a clear view of the uterus and fallopian tubes which makes it easier to diagnose and treat fertility issues.

Hysterosalpingogram

A hysterosalpingogram is an x-ray of the fallopian tubes and uterus. Dye is inserted in the fallopian tubes and the uterus. This makes the x-ray very clear so that blockages or even endometriosis can be identified.

Chapter 14

Getting Help To Conceive

In Vitro Fertilization

In Vitro Fertilization (IVF) refers to fertilization that takes place outside of the body. IVF is used when a woman suffers from blocked tubes or a man has a very low sperm count. In summary, it involves the harvesting of mature eggs and the subsequent fertilization of those eggs with sperm that has been collected. There are several steps involved in IVF. Each of them are discussed in further detail below.

The first step is ovulation induction, in this step, fertility drugs are used to stimulate the ripening of the egg. Egg development is monitored through the use of ultrasound which monitors the ovaries. Blood and urine tests are used to check hormone levels.

Secondly, an ultrasound is done to create a guide for the needle that will be inserted through the pelvic cavity in order to retrieve the eggs. The woman is usually sedated or put under local anesthesia to make the process of retrieval more comfortable. The removal of the eggs is called follicular aspiration. A few women may experience cramps after the eggs have been retrieved from their ovaries. This feeling often goes away after a day or so but some women report that they feel pressure in the ovaries several weeks after retrieval.

The third step involves the male partner who is asked to provide a sperm sample. This sperm sample is obtained by the collection of ejaculate.

The fourth step is called insemination, the sperm and eggs are put in incubators that provide the appropriate environment for fertilization. Sometimes, if there is considerably less chance for fertilization, a single sperm may be isolated and used in an attempt to achieve fertilization. Eggs are monitored constantly to ensure that cells are dividing and that fertilization is occurring. Once they are fertilized the eggs are known as embryos.

The fifth step is when the embryos are transferred to the uterus. A speculum is inserted in the vagina in order to get pass the cervix and into the uterus. A special number of embryos are then inserted in the uterus using a catheter. The process is painless for most women but there are exceptions and some women report mild discomfort. Finally, ultrasound and blood tests are done to see if implantation has occurred.

Artificial Insemination

Artificial insemination is a method that may help some couples who are struggling with infertility.

In this process, sperm is introduced into a woman's vagina. It can also be placed in the uterus or the fallopian tubes. However, the most popular way to do artificial insemination is the placing sperm into the uterus.

The success rate for artificial insemination is not as high as other more expensive and invasive methods. However, it has very few side effects which make it ideal for those who don't want to deal with more invasive and expensive methods.

It is the best choice for men whose sperm have motility issues and cannot swim to the egg on their own. In this case the sperm is introduced into the fallopian tubes. This technique may also work well for women who are suffering from endometriosis or other uterine abnormalities.

If a woman does not produce enough high quality cervical

fluid then it makes it very difficult for the sperm to swim to the egg. With artificial insemination, the sperm do not need the cervical fluid to help them swim to the egg, as they are introduced into the uterus without the help of the fluid.

Blood tests and ultrasounds are used to find out if the woman is ovulating before the procedure is done, also the woman's partner will be asked to abstain from sexual activity for two to five days to ensure that there is a high sperm count for the sample he will provide. Once the sample is collected, the sperm is washed in order to cleanse it of all harmful substances. A chemical is then mixed in with the sperm to find and isolate the ones that can swim the best, a centrifuge is then used to gather these sperm.

Once the sample is collected, it is introduced into the uterus via a catheter. This may cause some cramping and some light bleeding in some women but this often subsides quickly. Afterwards the woman is asked to lie down for about fifteen minutes. After this brief rest the procedure is complete and the woman can continue with her normal routine.

Conclusion

It is my hope that you have found this book helpful and that you now have a better understanding of your fertility. Hopefully, this guide will help you conceive quickly and assist you in dealing with any infertility issues you may be having, so that you can hold your bundle of joy as quickly as possible.

Wishing you lots of baby dust,

Simone Novelette

Like me on Facebook!

www.facebook.com/fertilityhaven

Other Titles By Simone Novelette

The Christian Wife: 9 Days Of Powerful, 10 Minute Devotions To Make You A Christ-Centered, Happy Wife

Made in United States
North Haven, CT
04 July 2023

38571328R00055